ERECTILE DYSFUNCTION CURE

HOW TO NATURALLY CURE ERECTILE DYSFUNCTION FOREVER

ADAM L. WISE

Table of Contents

Introduction... 1

Chapter 1: Understanding Erectile Dysfunction............. 3

Chapter 2: Erectile Dysfunction: Causes and Symptoms 7

Chapter 3: Improving Erectile Dysfunction Through Lifestyle Change... 13

Chapter 4: Improving Erectile Dysfunction Through Yoga.. 19

Chapter 5: Raw Juice Blends for Treating Erectile Dysfunction 23

Chapter 6: Kegel Exercise for Erectile Dysfunction 27

Chapter 7: Essential Oils for Erectile Dysfunction 31

Chapter 8: Intercourse Positions for Erectile Dysfunction.. 37

Chapter 9: How to Support Him in Dealing with Erectile Dysfunction 43

Chapter 10: Talk to Your Partner About Erectile
Dysfunction 47

Chapter 11: Erectile Dysfunction from a Female's
Perspective.. 51

Conclusion.. 55

Introduction

This book comprises proven measures and strategies on how to take full control of your sex life, the best way to treat erectile dysfunction, and proven steps to treat impotence naturally. Each step is discussed in chapters for better understanding.

Erectile dysfunction is a familiar condition among men, but it doesn't mean you can't do anything about it. Erectile dysfunction treatments need not be embarrassing or complicated. There are approaches and natural ways to overcome impotence.

Attempt these all-natural treatments and begin building your sexual self-confidence. You don't have to conceal your state. It can be treated, and you can have a healthy, happy sexual life. Everybody deserves it, and that includes you.

There is no better way to treat a condition like this. No need to experience pain, no gadgets to insert in your member, and no need to pay excessive physician fees.

These all-natural treatments are not only effective, they have become easy and discreet. Nobody needs to know you are getting treatment except you.

Chapter 1: Understanding Erectile Dysfunction

Erectile Dysfunction (ED), also known as impotence, can be a sexual disorder where the man struggles to get and keep an erection that is hard enough for sexual intercourse. Most men experience unexpected erectile dysfunction, especially when stressed, too tired, or under treatment. But regular erectile dysfunction has to be treated as it can be a sign of an actual health condition or emotional issues.

An erection can be difficult to attain as you age; however, it does not indicate that you will develop erectile dysfunction. The healthier you are, the better your sexual function.

Impotence problems are different from poor libido and ejaculation issues. To be certain, ED identifies the difficulties of achieving an erection and maintaining an erection. In some instances, a guy can have a healthy libido but struggle to keep an erection to make sexual activity possible.

This is a subject that most guys feel uncomfortable to speak about. However, it does exist and affects a large number of guys around the globe. But something many men do not know is why this happens or what can be achieved to fix or treat this issue.

Therefore, how can erections occur? The penis consists of two chambers called the corpora cavernosa, which is loaded with a spongy tissue called the corpus spongisum that encompasses the urethra. Erections begin when signals from the head and local nerves relax the muscles of the corpora cavernosa and then blood flows in and fills the sponge-like systems. This causes the penis to enhance and become hard.

Understanding this, what causes erectile dysfunction? A weak erection occurs when insufficient blood enters the corpora cavernosa. It may happen because of some harm to nerves or veins, which could be the result of a disease like diabetes, chronic alcoholism, or vascular and neurological disease. Other causes are: smoking, being overweight, side effects from drugs, or psychological factors like strain, anxiety, shame, depression, and fear of sexual failure.

This leads to the most crucial problem: How can these sexual conditions be treated? Physicians' suggestions can vary with each person. For some of them, some healthy changes in their lifestyle could be enough to solve their problem.

Chapter 2:
Erectile Dysfunction: Causes and Symptoms

Aging isn't the only cause of impotence problems. There are a number of causes that are unrelated to age, for example:

- Drug abuse

- Psychological causes (mental disorder, pressure or performance anxiety)

- Cavernosal problems including Peyronie's disease

- Kidney failure

- Diabetes mellitus

- Multiple sclerosis

- Smoking

- Excessive drinking

- Surgery

- Use of prescription drugs, for example: antidepressants, tranquilizers, and drugs for blood pressure

Prolonged drug abuse curbs the central nervous system and causes significant injury to blood vessels that will bring about impotence problems.

According to specialists, depression, tension, performance anxiety, and poor self-esteem may stop the process that creates an erection. These factors aggravate the problem in men whose erectile dysfunction is caused by something physical.

Some guys believe that drinking alcohol helps promote sex. However, heavy drinking could decrease the period you can sustain an erection since it is a depressant. To avoid this, reduce your alcohol use. Smoking causes plaque accumulation in blood vessels causing circulatory problems, which can lead to ED.

If you should be taking medication and you're having problems obtaining or keeping an erection, consult your doctor. Prescription drugs such as high blood pressure medicines, diuretics, antidepressants, antiepileptic, anti-panic, antihistamines, nonsteroidal anti-inflammatory drugs, medications for Parkinson's, antiarrhythmics, histamine H2 receptor antagonists, muscle relaxants, medications for prostate cancer, and chemotherapy medications may cause impotence problems.

Symptoms of Erectile Dysfunction

If you encounter any of these signs, consult your doctor for proper diagnosis.

- You suffer from late or premature ejaculation, have trouble obtaining an erection, or other sexual problems.

- You are struggling with heart disease or diabetes that's associated with ED.

- You experience other symptoms together with ED.

- Reduced libido and difficulty maintaining an erection.

Your family physician is the best place to begin as they already have your medical records.

The most known symptom of ED is not being able to achieve or sustain an erection during sexual activities with your partner. Other frequently mentioned symptoms are a failure of obtaining an erection during masturbation, failure of obtaining an erection even if there's obvious sexual desire, and lack of climax even with an extended lovemaking session.

ED is widespread and may be ranked differently according to severity of symptoms. Some may show a complete inability to get excited irrespective of the circumstances, while others will show partial inconsistent erections. Many men experience it and don't speak about it with their physicians until a vital case like a marital problem presents itself.

Causes of Erectile Dysfunction

There are lots of factors for the situation. The factors responsible might be mental or physical. However, many of the causes of erectile dysfunction are attributed to aspects of diabetes, age, physical condition, side effects of illicit drugs, performance pressure or anxiety, cardiac problems, and psychological factors. Other causes include the following:

1. Unhealthy lifestyle: Those who drink or smoke excessively may suffer from erectile dysfunction. It's been discovered that the intake of alcohol might reduce sperm count. Furthermore, excessive smoking may reduce your sex drive. Those who are on medications may also be affected by ED. Some studies have pointed out that guys who are overweight are at an increased risk of being affected by erectile dysfunction. Hence keeping a healthy lifestyle is very important to prevent erectile dysfunction.

2. Medicine: Erectile dysfunction may also be caused by unwanted side effects of any medications you are taking, especially those that are used to control your blood pressure. Other drugs that might be accountable for producing this condition are antihistamines, antidepressants, and cimetidine. There's also certain drugs that may affect the nervous system, which could lead to a blood vessel being damaged and causing permanent erectile dysfunction.

3. Surgery: Radical prostate and bladder surgeries can harm arteries and nerves that surround the penis. And this can cause ED. Other injuries that can cause erectile dysfunction are: penis injury and spinal cord injury, which may harm the arteries, muscles, nerves, and fibrous areas of the corpora cavernosa thus causing the condition.

4. Psychological: Psychological factors like stress, panic, shame, depression, and low self-esteem may also cause erectile dysfunction. In those situations, it's encouraged to seek psychiatric help.

Chapter 3:
Improving Erectile Dysfunction Through Lifestyle Change

Basic lifestyle changes will help improve erectile dysfunction. For males needing extensive treatment, lifestyle changes combined with other treatments can help them with more efficient, reliable, and faster results.

Quit Smoking

Quitting smoking is different for everybody. For some, going cold turkey is the best option. For others, they might need to be weaned off. However, you can start by steering clear of areas where you usually smoke. For those who wish to go cold turkey: set a date, discard all of your cigarettes, stay away from all smoking areas, and remain busy. For those who need to be weaned off: you can speak with your doctor about nicotine replacement therapy or a non-nicotine prescription.

Do not make it too hard on yourself. Go slowly, one day at a time. Desires are regular, but they'll disappear eventually. You may also get support by choosing to hitch a smoking cessation program that uses various techniques.

To make it easier, involve your family and friends. Ask them to keep you busy and tell them whenever you are tempted to possess another cigarette. Encouragements from friends and family help a whole lot in motivating one to move forward.

Limit Your Alcohol Intake

Nitric oxide is a chemical accountable for making erections and maintaining them. The central nervous system manages the release of this compound. Alcohol is a known depressant. If you drink a lot of alcohol, it depresses the central nervous system, which affects its operation and performance.

Because of this, the release of nitric oxide is also lowered, which can create impotence problems.

If you choose to drink, limit your alcohol intake to one to two glasses. If you suffer from alcohol addiction, you can start by consuming fresh fruit juice for 10–20 days, or whenever your cravings start. Pineapple juice, apple juice, orange juice, carrot juice, and bitter gourd juice are highly recommended. You may also join alcohol treatment programs to assist you to stop alcohol consumption faster.

If possible, keep a distance from friends and coworkers who drink a lot. If you need to go to a social gathering, have your spouse/friend/family member there or have your spouse/friend/family memeber call or text you from time to time to remind you never to take even one sip. It's going to be challenging, but with the help of your loved ones, it will become a lot easier.

Exercise

Whenever you exercise, your blood flow and blood pressure improves, which increases the levels of nitric oxide in your blood vessels. Exercise also helps increase production of testosterone naturally, an essential factor for sexual drive and erectile strength. Focus on light exercises for a few minutes. To obtain maximum benefits, exercise for at least 20–30 minutes every day.

Choose an exercise routine that increases blood flow and strengthens the pelvis and stomach area. Walking, running, and weight-bearing exercises are encouraged.

Eat Healthy

Everything you eat directly affects erectile dysfunction. Select a diet rich in whole grains, fruits, vegetables, and fish. If possible, decrease your intake of red meat and keep away from refined grains. It is very important to keep a healthy weight as reports show that men with a 42-inch waist are 50% more at risk of developing ED, compared with men with a 32-inch waist. Furthermore, obesity is related to diabetes and vascular disease, which can cause impotence problems.

To combat impotence, you need to eat foods that are rich in vitamin E. For example: leafy greens and wheat germ. Vitamin E improves blood circulation, which is essential for achieving an erection.

Zinc enhances testosterone levels. Foods full of zinc include sunflower seeds, chia seeds, pumpkin seeds, spinach, and lamb amongst others. Brazil nuts contain substantial quantities of selenium, which also boosts testosterone levels. For increased libido, eat some sesame seeds and watercress every day.

Follow a Sleep Schedule

Sleep loss affects testosterone levels in men. Low levels of sex hormones are connected to sexual dysfunctions. The body sticks to its internal clock to determine when it'll release certain hormones. Regular sleeping patterns ensure that your body gets a clear and consistent internal clock, making hormone secretions more effective.

Monitor Your Medications

If you must take medications for high blood pressure, heart conditions, depression, psychosis, hypertension, cancer, skin conditions, hormones, cholesterol, or baldness, and you suspect you have ED, you should consult your doctor. These drugs are known to cause impotence problems, and continued use can result in permanent ED.

You can find treatments for these conditions. However, you must consult expert professionals before trying one. Your doctor can also suggest alternative drugs, but should you choose to use alternative drugs, check with a specialist alternative physician for better understanding. Always consult your doctor before using any products as they could restrict other drugs.

Chapter 4:
Improving Erectile Dysfunction Through Yoga

Erectile dysfunction causes anguish for all men—and their partners. The good news is that it may be eradicated with yoga.

Yoga works on the whole person: body, mind, and spirit. As a result, it does not focus on one spot or one specific problem. This holistic approach ensures that the different contributory causes of a challenge are resolved (possibly the ones that you don't even know about), and you obtain other advantages to your health which come as unexpected gifts.

The different yoga postures provide a simple and normal approach to improving circulation, many of them being especially good for the genital and abdominal areas. Through regular yoga practices, the circulation of the body is increased and more air is distributed around every cell. Many longstanding conditions may be reduced or removed, and the natural recovery of the body is offered a fantastic increase. Ultimately, yoga helps the human body heal itself.

Typical yoga practice helps you increase energy. Unlike many exercise programs where one is normally exhausted by the end of the workout, yoga helps generate energy in the body. The ancient yogis called this "prana," the vital force. Whenever we possess a plentiful source of prana within the body, we feel alive, effective, and aware. This aliveness is contained in every cell and is a powerful drive to use during sex. Through the employment of meditative techniques, you can make use of an unlimited supply of this power.

Yoga also helps men by developing body-consciousness. A person can become aware of subtle changes in his body and consciously choose to use yogic processes to keep bodily energy or even to direct and keep blood flow.

The hypnotic aspect of yoga helps men let go of much of the emotional luggage which they bring to sex. For a few guys the pressure to perform creates real difficulties. Yoga helps men build self-confidence and inner poise.

Starting yoga isn't challenging, and a surprisingly large number of men practice already. It is common for men to attend yoga classes, and the good thing is that because it is a standard workout for people, nobody needs to know the details of why you attend.

Using pharmaceuticals as the answer to erectile dysfunction brings with it several negative effects. The benefit of yoga is the fact that all of its effects are positive—great all-around health, youthfulness, and peace of mind.

Chapter 5:
Raw Juice Blends for Treating Erectile Dysfunction

Many people have tried juicing for weight loss, detox, and as a remedy for various conditions. Selected fruits and vegetables contain antioxidants and nutrients that increase production of nitric oxide and increase blood circulation, which is why you can also go on a liquid diet for erectile dysfunction problems. Listed below are numerous fluid combinations you can make at home to deal with your ED.

Carrot Cucumber Beet Juice

Ingredients

10 oz. carrots

3 oz. cucumbers

3 oz. beets

Directions

1. Cut the fruits into smaller pieces.

2. If utilizing a juicer, spot fruits within the chute and liquid based on manufacturer's guidelines.

3. If employing a blender, blend ingredients until smooth.

4. Drink once each morning and once in the evening before bedtime.

Banana Kale Pineapple

Ingredients

1 medium banana

4 kale leaves

1 cup pineapple chunks

Directions

1. Place all components withing the blender and pulse until smooth.

2. You might include 4–5 ice cubes to help make the drink thinner and make it cooler.

3. Drink twice daily.

Pomegranate Juice

Ingredients

3 pomegranates

1 teaspoon honey

Directions

1. Wash pomegranates and cut into smaller pieces to fit the chute of your juice extractor. Don't remove the skin or vegetables.

2. Juice as usual.

3. Put in a teaspoon of honey if you would like it sweeter.

4. Drink twice every day.

Watermelon Pomegranate Juice

Ingredients

½ medium watermelon

2 pomegranates

Directions

1. You need to use a blender or a juicer.

2. Slice the fruits into smaller slices and blend or juice. Remember to remove and discard the watermelon rind as it could make your liquid bitter and bad.

3. You can refrigerate any leftovers and drink at a later time.

4. If refrigerated, it might last up to 3 days.

These juice combinations are all-natural and don't include any artificial ingredients. Besides treating erectile dysfunction, these juice combinations also help keep your body healthier; you're killing two birds with one stone.

Plus, these juice blends taste awesome. You can combine them in your diet, and you won't even notice that you're going through an ED treatment. Also, you can combine these liquid blends with other alternative ED treatments including yoga, exercise, and others. It's very safe and effective, too.

Chapter 6:
Kegel Exercise for Erectile Dysfunction

Kegel exercises are recommended for women who just gave birth to restore muscle tone in their pelvic region. However, current studies suggest that Kegel exercise can also be beneficial for men with erectile dysfunction and premature ejaculation problems. Furthermore, Kegel exercise also enhances the quality of orgasms, bringing on a better sexual experience.

How to do a Kegel exercise

1. Identify your pelvic floor or lower pelvis. You can do this by preventing your pee midstream. The muscle that you clench to stop your urine is the muscle that you might want to strengthen.

2. Press your pelvic floor muscles and maintain it for 5 seconds. Breathe and relax.

3. Repeat after 10 seconds. You can start by performing 10 rounds and steadily increase while you go along.

4. Try this Kegel exercise in numerous positions such as standing, resting on your joints, and lying down.

Another Kegel exercise you can look into is pressing the muscles around your anus. Do that just like you are stopping your chair from venturing out. Stay in that position for 5 seconds while breathing then relax the muscles. Repeat around 10 times and increase as you go on.

These Kegel exercises can be carried out everywhere. You can do it at home, at the office, as well as when you are driving, observing a film, or relaxing in your bath.

Premature ejaculation (PE) can be a very common sexual dysfunction present in almost half of all men. The emotional effects of the discomfort and humiliation caused by this disorder are huge and more often than not go untreated. Premature ejaculation might be successfully treated in your home without using any mind or body-altering drugs and at almost no cost. The condition is essentially created early-on by incorrect teenage sexual behaviors and later by pressure and emotional anxiety. It is not the result of any medical or physiological problem. The solution is to create a strategy to reprogram the mind and body to manage your sexual sensations. With appropriate practice and dedication you'll be amazed by the outcome.

The pubococcygeus muscle, or PC muscle, forms part of the pelvic floor and is in charge of the movement of semen and urine in men. In order to prevent premature ejaculation, one should define their PC muscle and thus acquire control of their sexual endurance.

To strengthen this muscle, attempt to quit the flow of urine the next time you are in the bathroom. The big advantage of doing Kegels is the fact that they can be performed anywhere and no one would know.

Chapter 7:
Essential Oils for Erectile Dysfunction

Physical and psychological factors can also influence erectile dysfunction. Essential oils can help reduce impotence by stimulating blood flow and taking care of any underlying psychological issues you're experiencing.

Essential oils have already been useful for ages to cure many health problems and impotence isn't an exception.

Below are some essential oils which will help cure erectile dysfunction.

Basil: The smell of basil arouses sexual instincts. Additionally, it calms down stress.

Black Pepper: It relieves exhaustion and melts self-doubt. It restores sexual energy by warming the human body and alleviating emotions.

Cardamom: Due to its aphrodisiac properties, cardamom is employed to boost sexual desire and libido. It contains cineole, a substance that influences the central nervous system.

Cedarwood: This oil arouses sensual feelings and improves sexual response. It also calms concerns and fears regarding sex.

Clary Sage: This herb supports greater sleep, reduces anxiety, and relieves depression. It also increases sexual interest and arouses sexual thoughts. It is best employed for impotence caused by mental elements because it opens negative feelings and removes inhibitions.

Ginger: It is an aphrodisiac. It stimulates sexual desires and warms the human body, thus, increasing libido.

Geranium: It relaxes the muscles and helps relieve stress, fatigue, and anxiety. It is also an aphrodisiac, antidepressant, and antioxidant.

Jasmine: Its nice, floral scent is very intoxicating and relaxing. It's also an aphrodisiac. It warms your body and promotes deep sleep. Also, it burns up anger and disappointment.

Juniper: This essential oil is better for ED on account of emotional and mental elements. It removes relationship insecurities, arouses love and sex, and promotes self-confidence.

Lavender: Its flowery, intoxicating, sweet scent arouses sexual emotions. In a report about male reaction to aromatherapy, lavender is demonstrated to increase penile blood flow by 40%. Additionally, it wards off stress and anxiety.

Neroli: This oil can be an aphrodisiac, and it effectively releases anxiety regarding sex.

Rose: It increases intimacy in couples. It also advances the sensation of love and dispels fear of intimacy.

Sandalwood: It stimulates delicate emotions and refreshes the mind and body. It's also an aphrodisiac and assists with frigidity and impotence.

Vetiver: This oil reduces concerns and tensions. It is sexually stimulating and strengthens sexual desires.

Ylang-ylang: It's used as an aphrodisiac. It revitalizes overall power, relaxes the body, and encourages soothing sleep. It also relieves depression and stress.

You can add these essential oils to your bath water or rub them into your genitals. Be sure you combine them with a carrier oil before using as a massage oil or immediately using on your skin.

Listed here are essential oil mixtures for treating erectile dysfunction.

Blend 1

20 drops basil
15 drops clary sage
10 drops ylang-ylang
1 drop clove
1 drop patchouli
1 oz. jojoba oil or coconut oil

Combine all oils in a glass bottle. You may use it directly on your genitals and massage some on your pelvic area. You can even add this mixture to your bath.

Blend 2

30 drops clary sage

30 drops fennel

20 drops sage

10 drops yarrow

5 drops peppermint

Mix oils carefully. To use directly on your skin, add 1 oz. jojoba oil, sesame seed oil, or coconut oil. You can even use this mix in your diffuser, preferably one hour or 3 minutes before having sex. You can also add this mix to your warm bath. Mix oils in 1 tbsp. honey and mix in your warm bathwater.

Blend 3

30 drops geranium

30 drops rosewood

15 drops ylang-ylang

10 drops myrrh

10 drops black pepper

Combine the oils in 1 oz. jojoba oil and use it to massage your top, back, and pelvic area. You can even use it on your genitals. You may also include this blend in your warm bath.

Blend 4

10 drops rosewood

1 drop sandalwood

8 drops clary sage

6 drops thyme

6 drops ylang-ylang

4 drops coriander

Mix all oils and add to your diffuser or light. Use about an hour before bedtime. You may also add this combination to your bath. Utilize it in the morning and the evening for maximum benefits.

Some people have extremely sensitive skin. Before you use any of these mixes directly on your skin, be sure to do a skin patch test. Apply a small amount of your chosen mix on your hand and dab it at the trunk of your palm. Wait for one hour and look for any responses. If you have none, you can use the blend safely for your diffuser, shower, or topical use.

Chapter 8:
Intercourse Positions for Erectile Dysfunction

Erectile difficulties aren't rare, and they're nothing to worry about when they just happen once in a while. If you have problems in 50% of the circumstances where you wish to have sex, you might consider erectile dysfunction a condition. A topic that was long discussed in the medical world is if there are particular sexual positions for erectile dysfunction that can help a man suffering from this condition. Those experiencing impotence problems need to be aware of the truth that it might take a lot more than changing their sexual position to solve their problem.

Blood flow to the penis accounts for an erection and physicians agree that sexual positions involving numerous "acrobatics" might not be appropriate for those suffering from ED simply because they might reduce the blood flow to the region. For some time, the medical community decided that the greatest sexual position for erectile dysfunction is with a girl at the top, but today doctors are not so sure about it. Nowadays, it's largely decided that sexual positions for ED depend on the couple. What might work for two people might not be comfortable or enjoyable for others. Some think the missionary position is best for men suffering from erectile dysfunctions, while others still feel a woman on top is best.

Regardless of the sexual position for impotence problems a couple considers most appropriate, a much better approach in treating this problem would be to stop focusing on the sexual act so much and just be mindful of the intimate occasion with your partner. Communication and intimacy can help you discover the best sexual position for ED for the both of you, or even the position that will bring the most pleasure for you.

Only thinking about how you may react to sex brings added stress and can affect your efficiency instead of centering on growing your partner's pleasure and developing a comfortable and enjoyable atmosphere for both of you. There's no such thing as a general sexual position for impotence problems. Everyone has to learn what is best for them, and a good way of doing this is by increasing intimacy between you and your partner. You may also try some herbal supplements to heal this issue forever.

Unique sexual positions have been identified to provide more control to men who are suffering from erectile dysfunction. But make no mistake there's no general rule for this.

Relax mentally entirely before you have sex. If one is emotionally affected by his past episodes of disappointment, nothing might help him. Think that you are healthy and can do it as effective as anyone else instead of thinking what went wrong last time. Sex isn't all about reproductive organs. It is about the entire body. Relax and stimulate your partner by kisses, hugs, caresses, kneading, and expressing nice words in their ears. This will turn them on and will help you in take them to climax before you reach yours.

Lady on the top position has been utilized by several men who have a tendency to lose their erection during sex. In this situation, you can relax in a comfortable position, and it will be your partner making the movements.

Within this position, men can stimulate their partner and also enjoy and keep their excitement. This will ultimately aid in keeping you involved in the work emotionally while allowing you to maintain your erection.

Face-to-face position also assists in countering erectile dysfunction during sex. Many couples find this sexual position effective in handling erectile dysfunction. While the man is in a sitting position, his partner sits in his lap facing him. The man might help to ensure that his partner can put their feet around his waist. This situation enables the male to penetrate his partner better. For those who have made your partner aware of your problem, then your partner can ensure that your enjoyment stays intact to keep up the amount of blood in your genitals. Make sure that that you don't sit on a hard floor while trying this position.

Approaching your partner from behind while they're lying sideways and penetrating them by bending their upper leg can be an effective sexual situation for erectile dysfunction. That is also a position that won't cause overexertion and it gives pleasure to both parties, thus keeping up the levels of excitement. Apart from this, it's easy for the guy to maintain his penetration even though his stiffness is decreasing.

Bear in mind these are simply guidelines. These sex positions may or may not work for you. Locate a position you are comfortable with and are highly in control. For a better lovemaking experience, incorporate the proposed treatments within this book and find out which works best for you.

Furthermore, lovemaking is extremely personal and close. Make it extra special by adding more energy into it. Perhaps you can diffuse some sensually stimulating essential oils and add some candles and flowers. This may not just make your partner feel more unique; it will also help them feel engrossed. Likewise, once you see your partner happy, it gives you more confidence and will make you more sexually aroused.

Finally, you must be honest with your partner. You must communicate your issue with them. Moreover, ask them what excites them sexually. Knowing this will assist you to keep them happy and satisfied during sex without shattering your confidence.

Chapter 9:
How to Support Him in Dealing with Erectile Dysfunction

Whenever a girl first finds that her partner has erectile dysfunction, it could be very damaging. Before learning about his situation, you might have been wondering what has gone wrong with your sexual relationship. A wide range of issues may go through your mind. *Is he bored having sex with me? Am I not desirable anymore?* Worse, it might take a while for him to be able to tell you the truth. Up until he confesses what's wrong, he has probably tried his best to handle the challenge by himself because he was afraid of your answer or embarrassed that ED makes him feel less manly. He may avoid intimacy that could lead to sex, including trying not to touch you or going to bed straight away without sex. Each time you ask, he may have said nothing was wrong, or he was just exhausted or didn't feel like it. Since you have realized the problem, you need to support him as best as you can. There are certainly a few things you can do.

First of all, you need to learn about erectile dysfunction. Find out as much as you possibly can. You can look up information on the Internet, learn from health guides, as well as talk with an expert who can tell you everything about ED and probably how you should help your partner. When you have obtained adequate information and knowledge about ED, you'll be able to assist your partner and assist him to deal with it in the best possible way. Whether he has started treatment or continues to be looking for a remedy, the two of you need to discuss what kind of treatment will fit him best and make you both feel comfortable. However, if that method doesn't work, then it is time for him to try another strategy that may not be as comfortable but gives better results. Tell him that you're certain that he'll be able to cure his ED, and there are lots of different methods, that if one fails, he shouldn't worry. The next thing you must do is accompany him to visit a doctor, as long as he does not mind your presence. This may show him that you support him. As an unhealthy lifestyle also adds to ED, you should also encourage him to keep a healthy lifestyle, for example being on a wholesome diet, helping him quit smoking, reduce drinking, and exercising more frequently. The most important thing you must do is to tell him that ED doesn't make him less of a man in your eyes and that it is not an unusual problem, which many guys, even younger ones, also suffer from the same problem. When he is feeling frustrated, be there for him, or give him space so he can take care of his own frustration.

It may take time to overcome erectile dysfunction. Have patience with the treatment process and also help him to have patience, too. Regarding your sex life, both of you do not need to feel stressed simply because of his condition. There are many things you can do to keep the spice in your sex life. Research how couples with this same problem can still have fun in bed, and discover other things related to it that you may not have known before. Your sex life can still be exciting as you wait for his treatment to show results.

Chapter 10:
Talk to Your Partner About Erectile Dysfunction

It is very important that you speak to your partner about erectile dysfunction if it's something you are experiencing. Although erectile dysfunction is talked about openly in today's community, it might nevertheless be an awkward topic to you and your partner. Lots of men do not discuss the situation with their companion since they feel embarrassed that they cannot perform. It is important that you know the reality of erectile dysfunction, and that you include your partner in the procedure of coping with it.

Discussing the topic can be hard. Sometimes you simply do not know where to begin or what to talk about. That's okay. There are several different ways you may approach and talk about it. The first thing you'll want to do is to choose a way to approach the subject that is comfortable for you. If your partner introduces the topic instead of you, don't shut them down or feel like they are attacking you. Listen and make them feel comfortable.

Though you may feel attacked if your partner asks you about it first, you must realize that your partner also wants openness and support. Sometimes impotence problems are equally as hard on the partner as the person experiencing it. Your partner may be blaming themselves for not being attractive enough, or they might think that you are avoiding sex because of your feelings for them. Your partner needs to be assured that this is simply not the event and that you need their assistance as you take care of the matter.

You should also know the value of emotional intimacy. Some sex therapists propose that you take a break from sexual intimacy while you focus on coping with the erectile dysfunction, and instead focus on the emotional intimacy. While erectile dysfunction is often the result of an actual condition, additionally it may be the effect of an emotional problem. Including your partner in emotional intimacy can help if that's the case.

It is essential that both you and your partner realize that erectile dysfunction is a serious problem—one that you should consult your doctor about. Don't attempt to treat impotence problems on your own, as there are so many causes and explanations why you could be experiencing it.

The most significant thing as far as your relationship can be involved, is the fact that you keep the communication open. Share your feelings with your partner and ask for their feelings in return. Offer love and help, and you will almost certainly get that in return.

Chapter 11:
Erectile Dysfunction from a Female's Perspective

Impotence might have significant effects in the life of a woman than we normally consider it to be. Impotence problems can shatter a woman's life and keep her in emotional shambles. Sex is the sacred marriage of two physical systems, with the spiritual bonding of two minds and individuals into a single entity; it is all about mutual sharing, satisfying one's partner in the course of satisfying oneself. While each one of the parties fails to perform its part, the connection can gradually weaken, thus resulting in the pair having to pay a heavy price.

We keep talking about impotence or impotence problems only from a guy's point of view, never for a minute pondering over what the feminine partner could be feeling. Typically, of ED, the feminine counterpart often winds up emotionally damaged. Men with a hurt pride typically begin acting in strange ways to cover-up their frustrations on their loss of manliness. Occasionally, he even becomes severe with his partner, prepared to attack with lethal fangs. Instead of asking her for help or discussing the issue with her, he gradually drifts far from her for reasons only he knows.

Well, what do you expect from the woman, his companion? She may sometimes transfer to her shell and develop into a recluse, or at best rebel and get on with living just how she knows best.

The sexual build up in a lady before sex has more to do with thoughts than just basic physical cravings; it is a slow but steady progress that reaches its crescendo with a beautiful climax. Researchers show that many women fail to get an orgasm, even when their male partners have no erectile problems. Just imagine the gravity of the situation, when a person is hopelessly impotent.

Ladies feel neglected when men try to escape due to erectile dysfunction. Like any sexual partner, she has every right to know about the issue; and as a life partner, she's entitled to at least some amount of trust from her man. If he fails to share his sexual problem with her, she may slowly lose her trust in the relationship.

Why do men fail to recognize the fact that women can reach an orgasm even without penetrative sex? Together, the man and woman can come up with novel ideas of enjoying the pleasures of sex that will not necessarily require the penis. Men never realize that they hurt a woman by keeping their sexual problems to themselves.

Sometimes, the dissatisfaction and the annoyance of a barren sexual patch in their life may push her to the degree of looking for different partners to satisfy her basic instincts of love, care, and sex. The strong-willed might try every possible way to put the zing back in their relationship, the more rebellious might move away and could even file for legal separation, and it should not come as a surprise if some consider committing suicide.

But a lot still sits on the man. A woman could always be ready to have him back in her arms, and work together for constructive approaches to overcome his erectile problems. Guys need to understand the challenges women have. The open-minded approach of a man can build up the trust and faith necessary for the lovers to defeat the nightmares of erectile dysfunction.

Conclusion

Thank you again for purchasing this book!

I hope this book was able to help you address and assume control of your impotence problems. Don't let your relationship dwindle. Impotence problems could be addressed and managed using different strategies which are not only easy but also affordable. These solutions do not need to be uncomfortable or artificial. Natural remedies are often the most effective because they do not have adverse side effects, and they feature a lot of health benefits.

The next step is to maintain your body and relationship by following easy steps to treat and cure erectile dysfunction that has been outlined in this book. These solutions are simple to follow, and they could easily be done at home. Moreover, these cures don't simply address impotence; they also improve your sexual health and overall well-being.

Finally, if you enjoyed this book, then I'd like to ask you for a favor. Would you be kind enough to leave a review for this book on Amazon? It'd be greatly appreciated!

Thank you and good luck!

Other books by Adam L. Wise

The Power of Habits
Creating Habits For Success to Change Your

Become successful and achieve everything you ever wanted by creating new small habits. If you fill your everyday lives with habits that lead you to success, you'll eventually see yourself in a position that you have dreamed of, a position wherein you are free to do anything you want and earn the money you want.

Feng Shui Secrets
The Ultimate Guide to Improve Your Health, Wealth and Relationships

Feng shui will be your helping hand for your health, wealth and relationships. True feng shui is no longer a mystery; it is simple and un-demanding. It is not just about planning gigantic buildings and momentous architecture. It is as simple as setting your living room in a positive and helpful way. Just give this book a read and you will be convinced of the miracles feng shui can do for you!

Crystals
Crystal Healing and Crystal Magic for Health, Love and Money

If you want to learn ancient healing and magical secrets, you should learn how to use crystals for multiple purposes in order to obtain any desired result in your life. Consult this book and you will find the answers to each and every query you have.

www.ingramcontent.com/pod-product-compliance
Lightning Source LLC
Chambersburg PA
CBHW060646290526
45793CB00001B/415